This Book Belongs To:

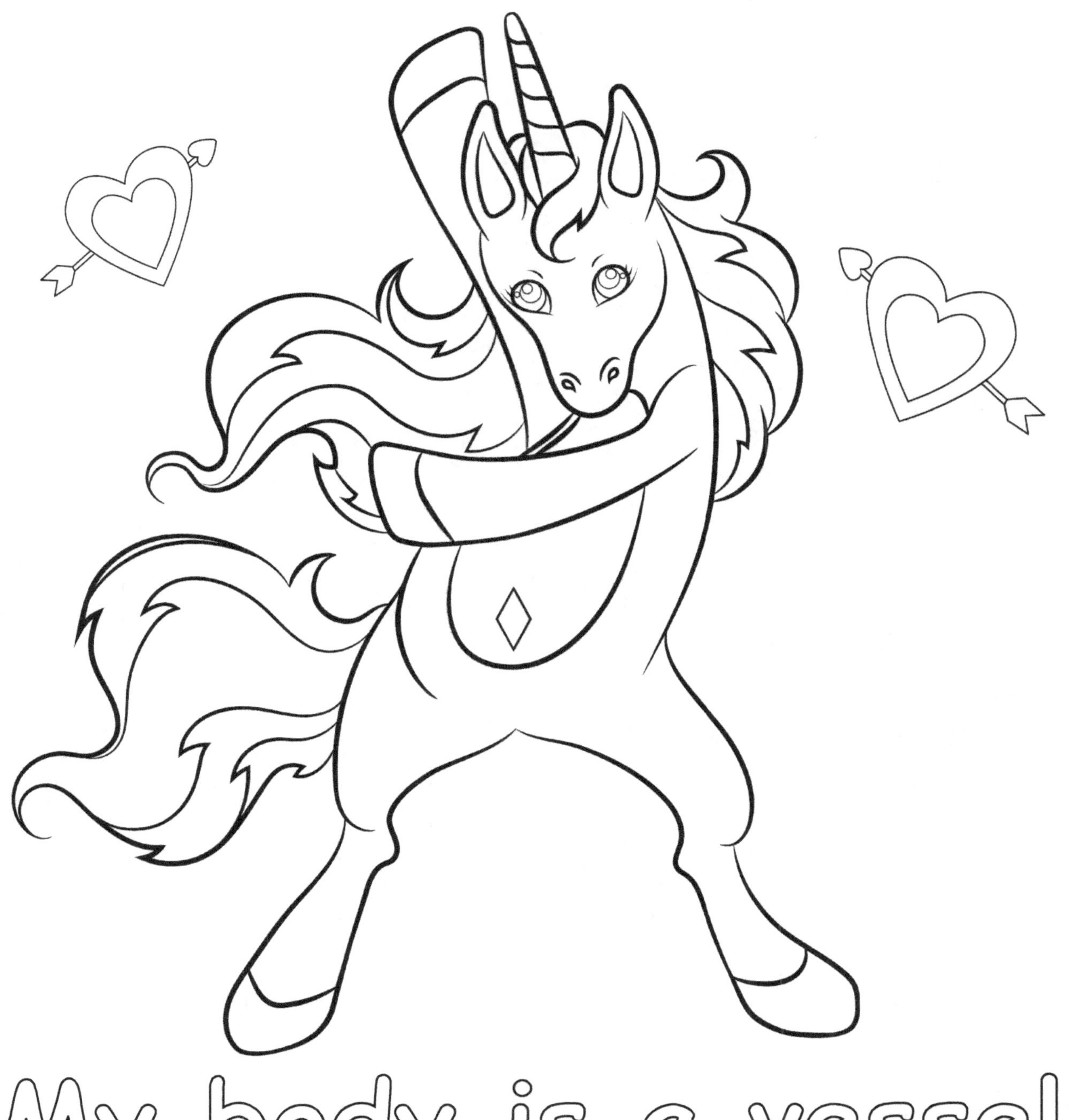

My body is a vessel for my awesomeness

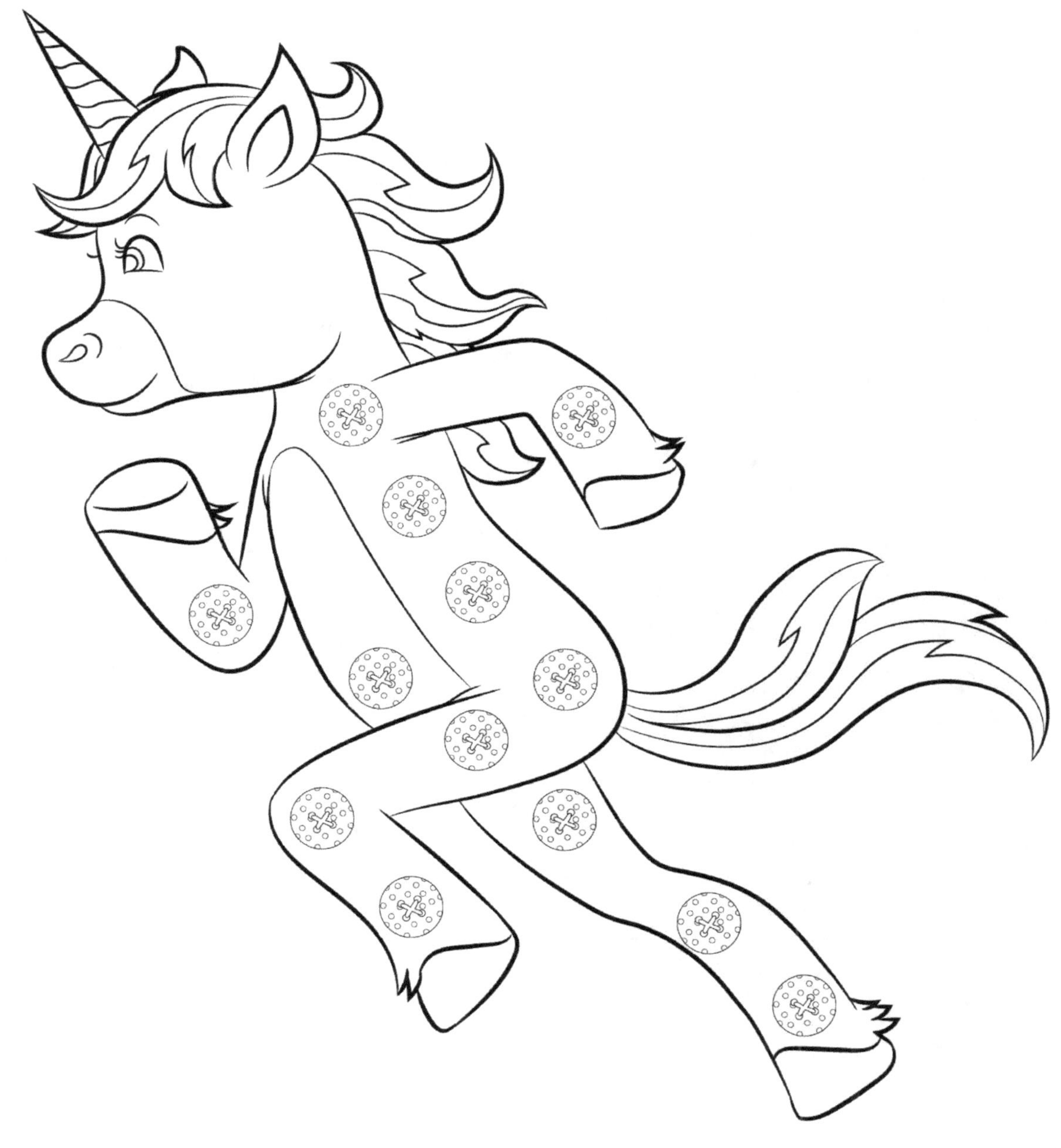

My body is strong

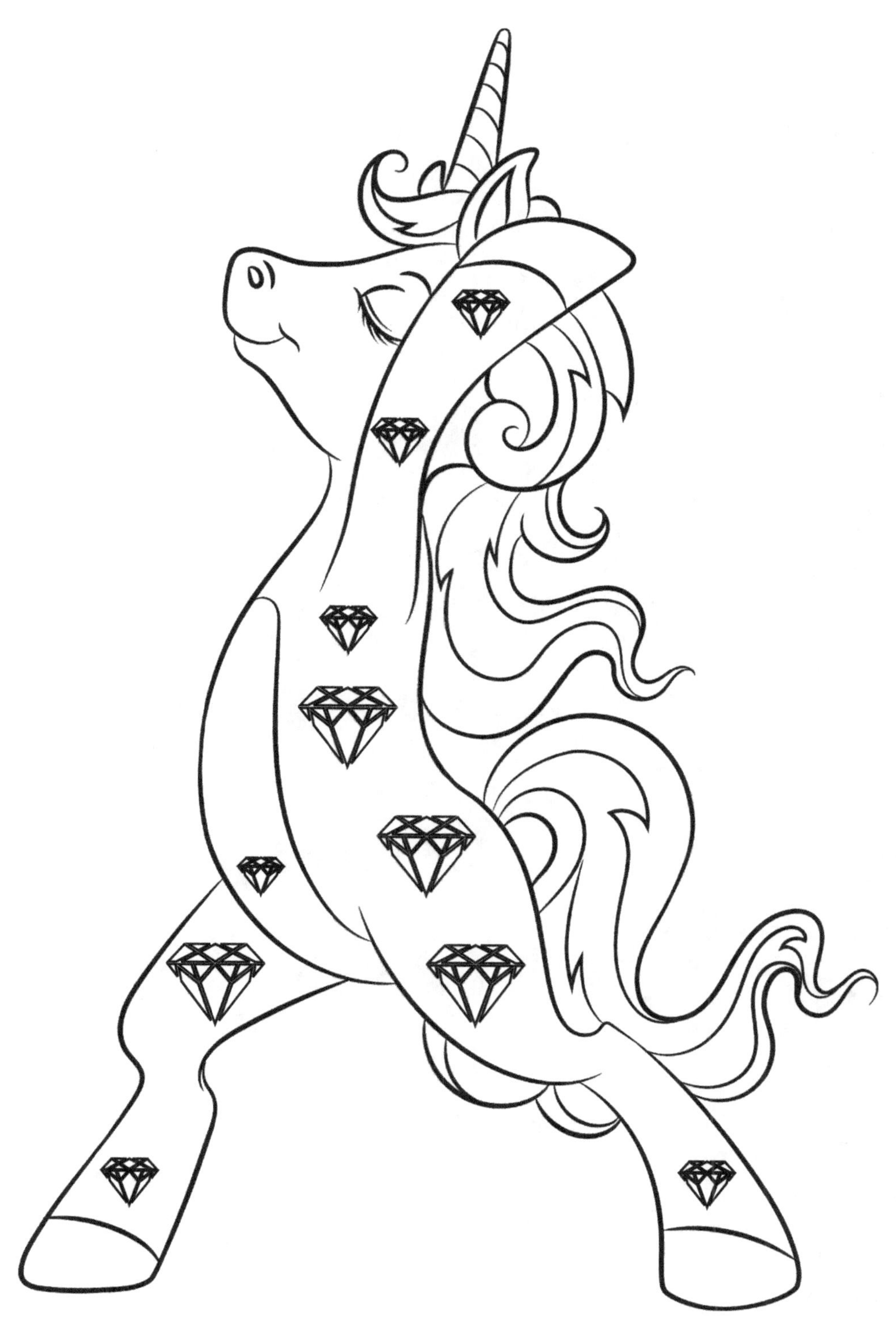

My body takes care of
me and i take care of it

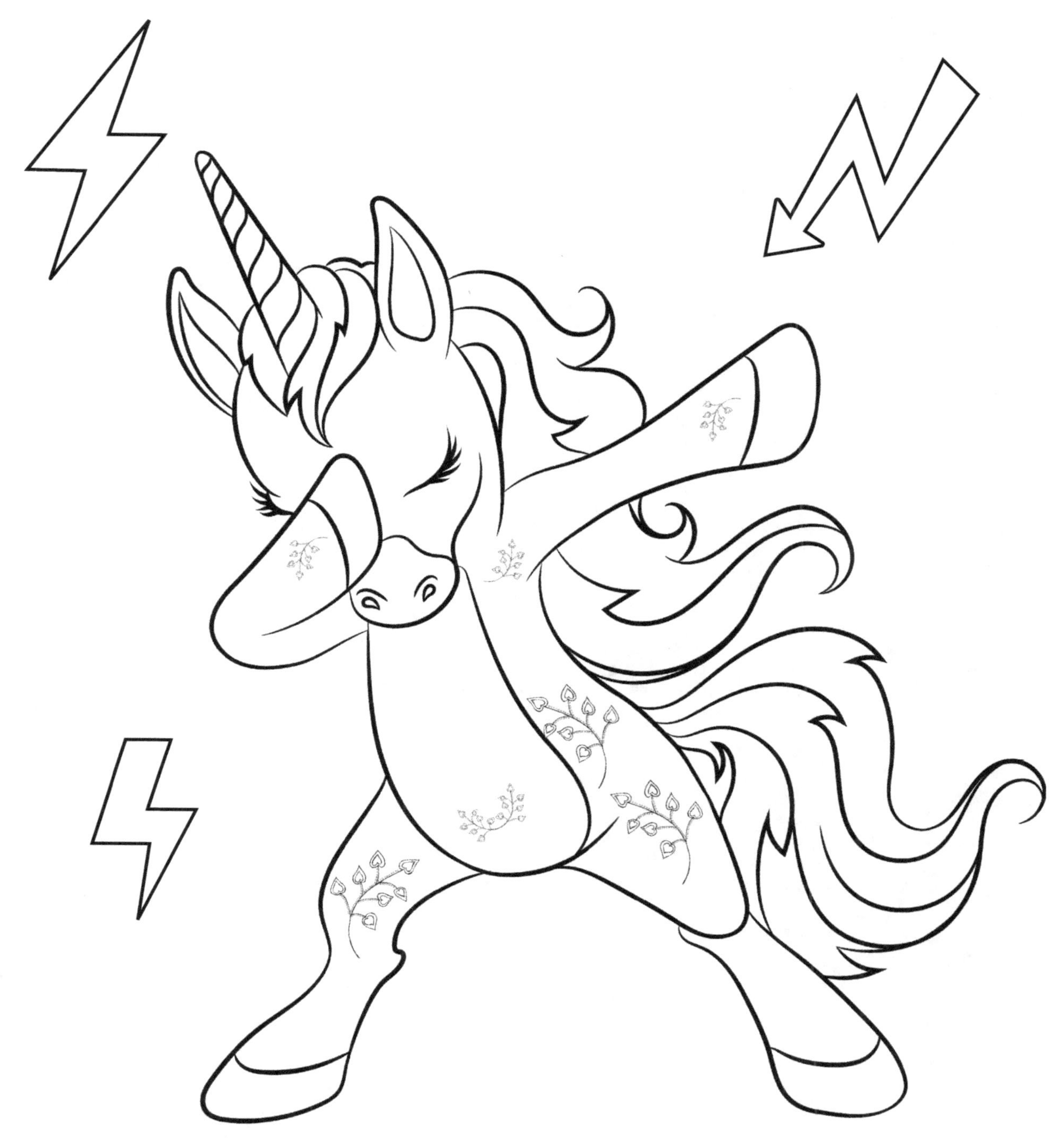

My body is perfectly unique

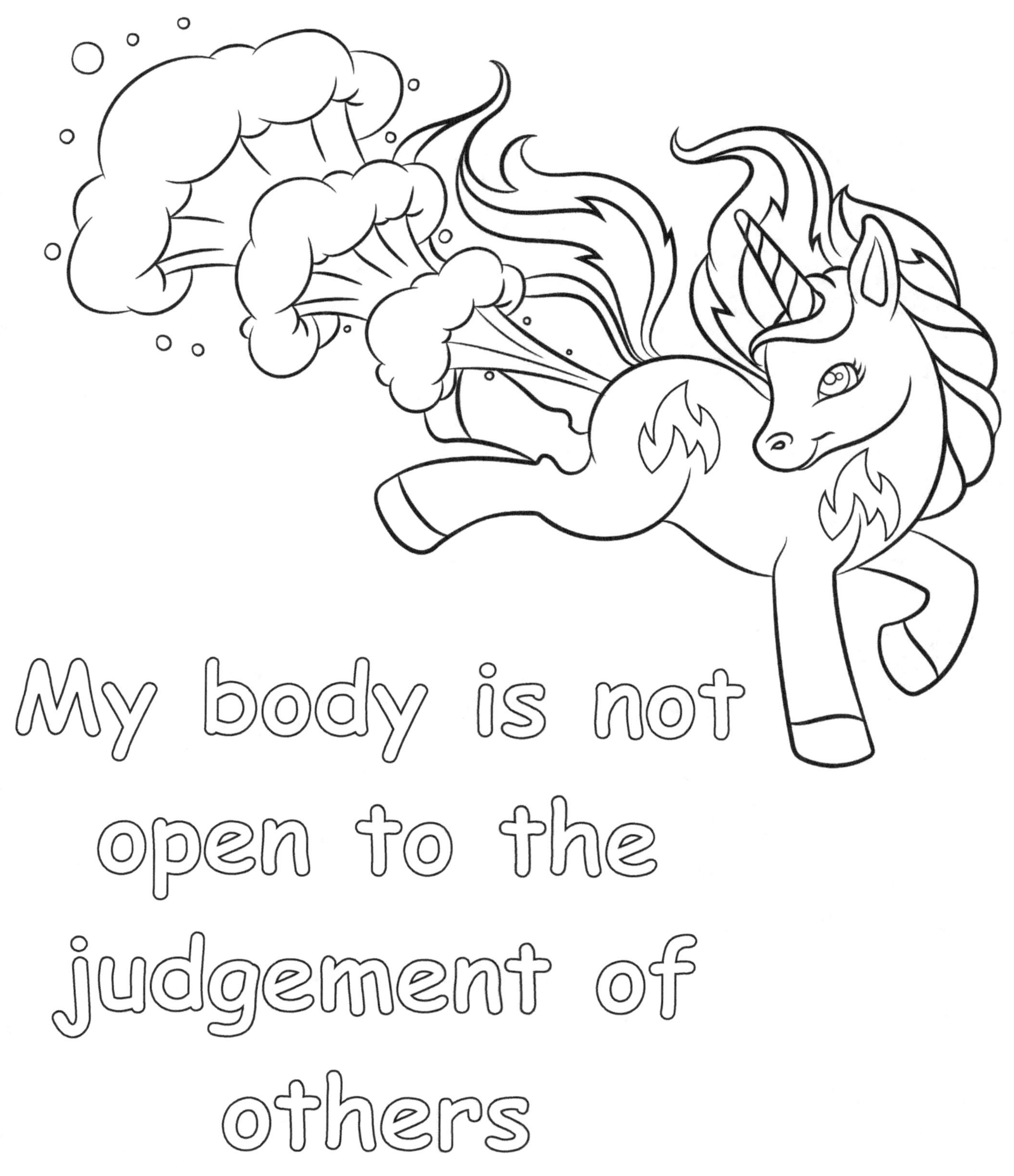

My body is not open to the judgement of others

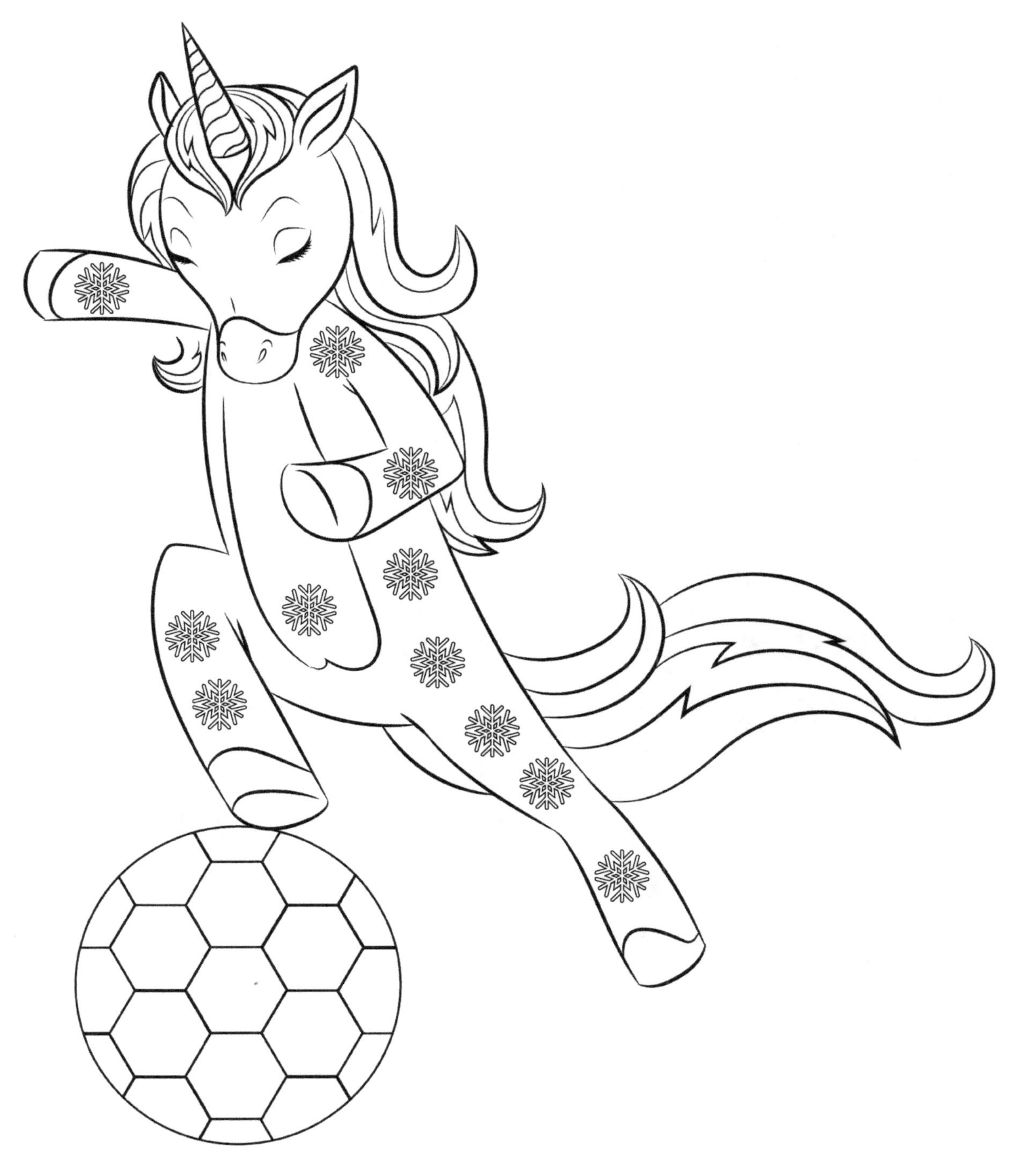

My body is athletic

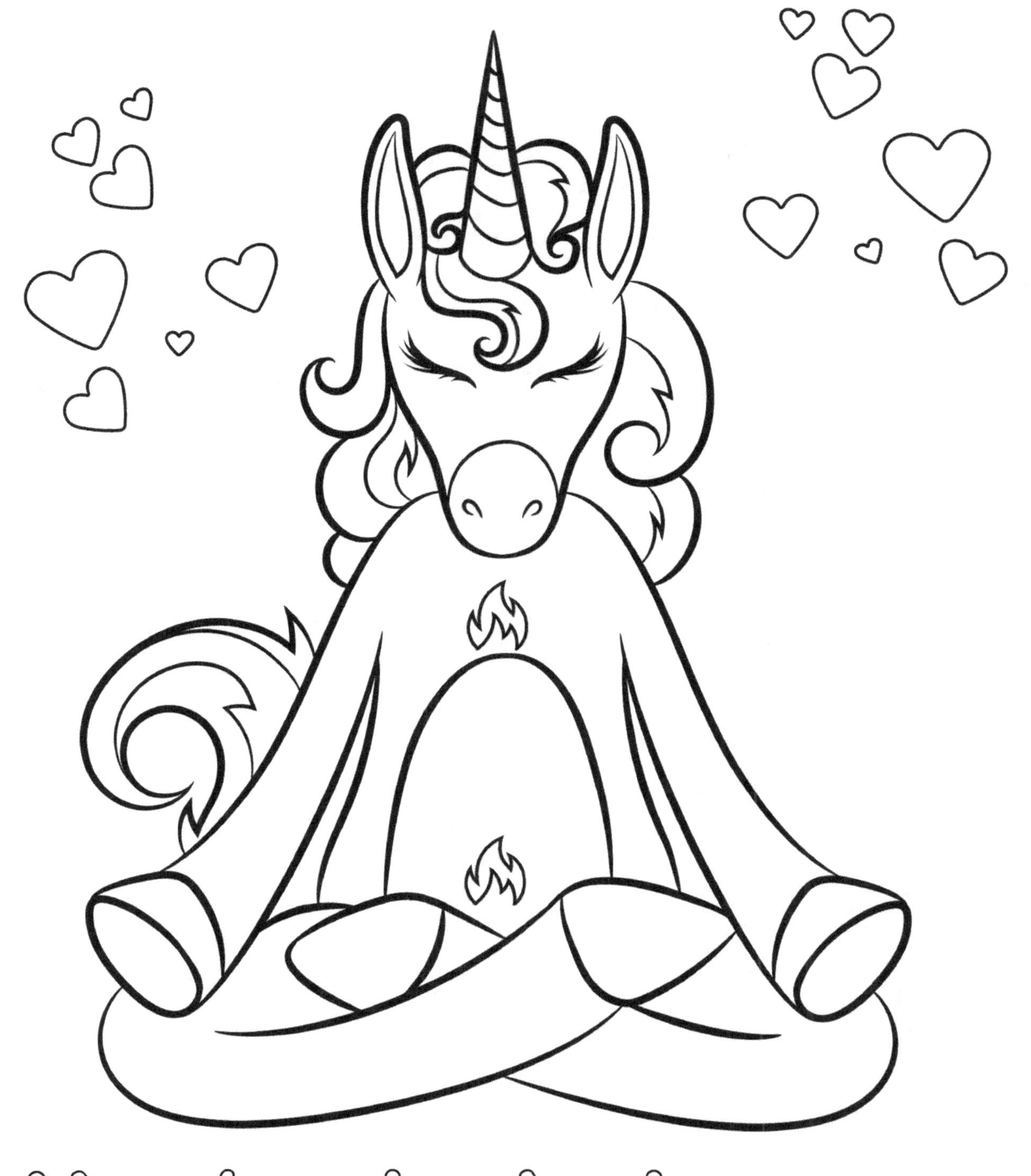

My body helps me
feel happy and loved

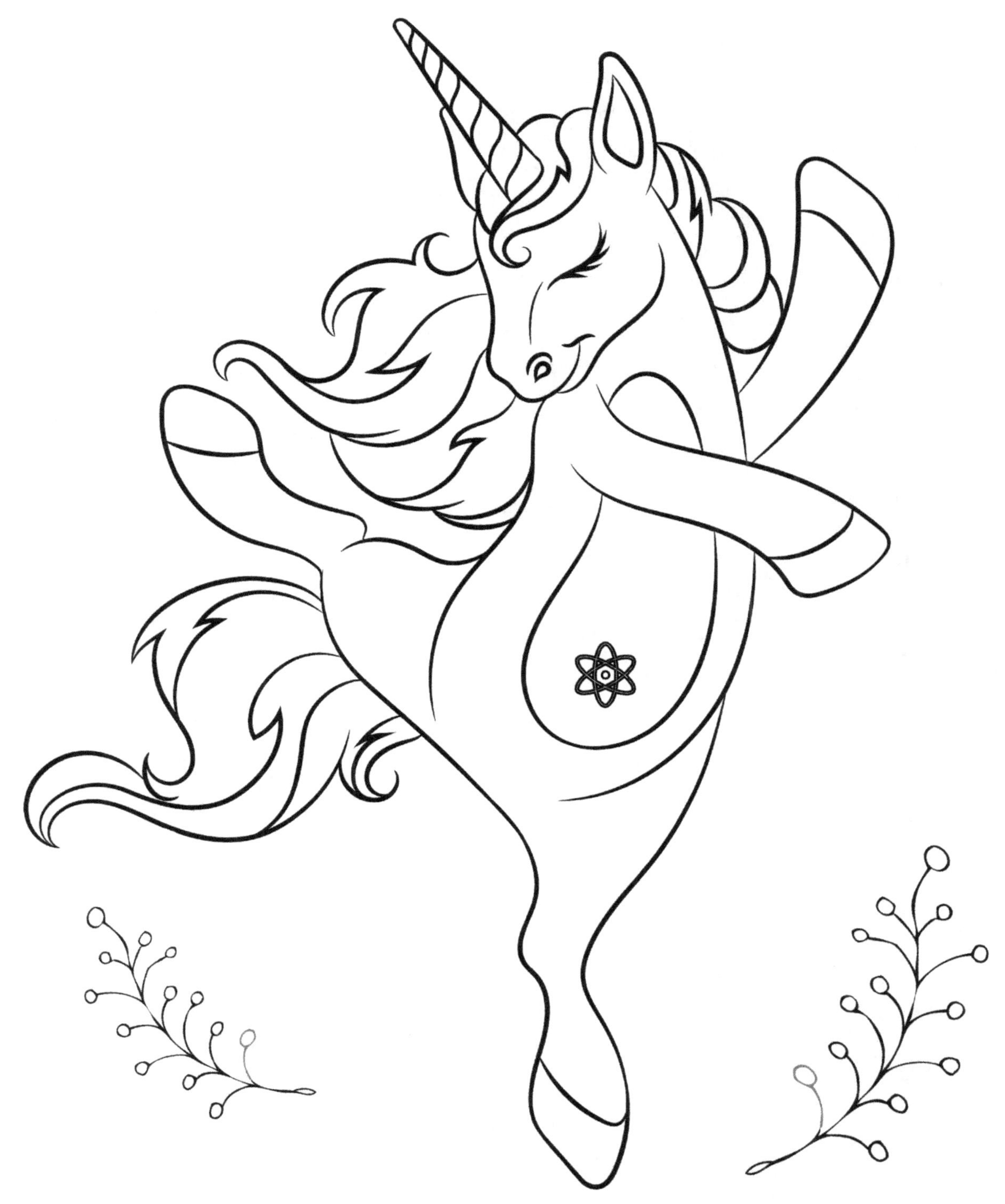

My body is capable
of great things

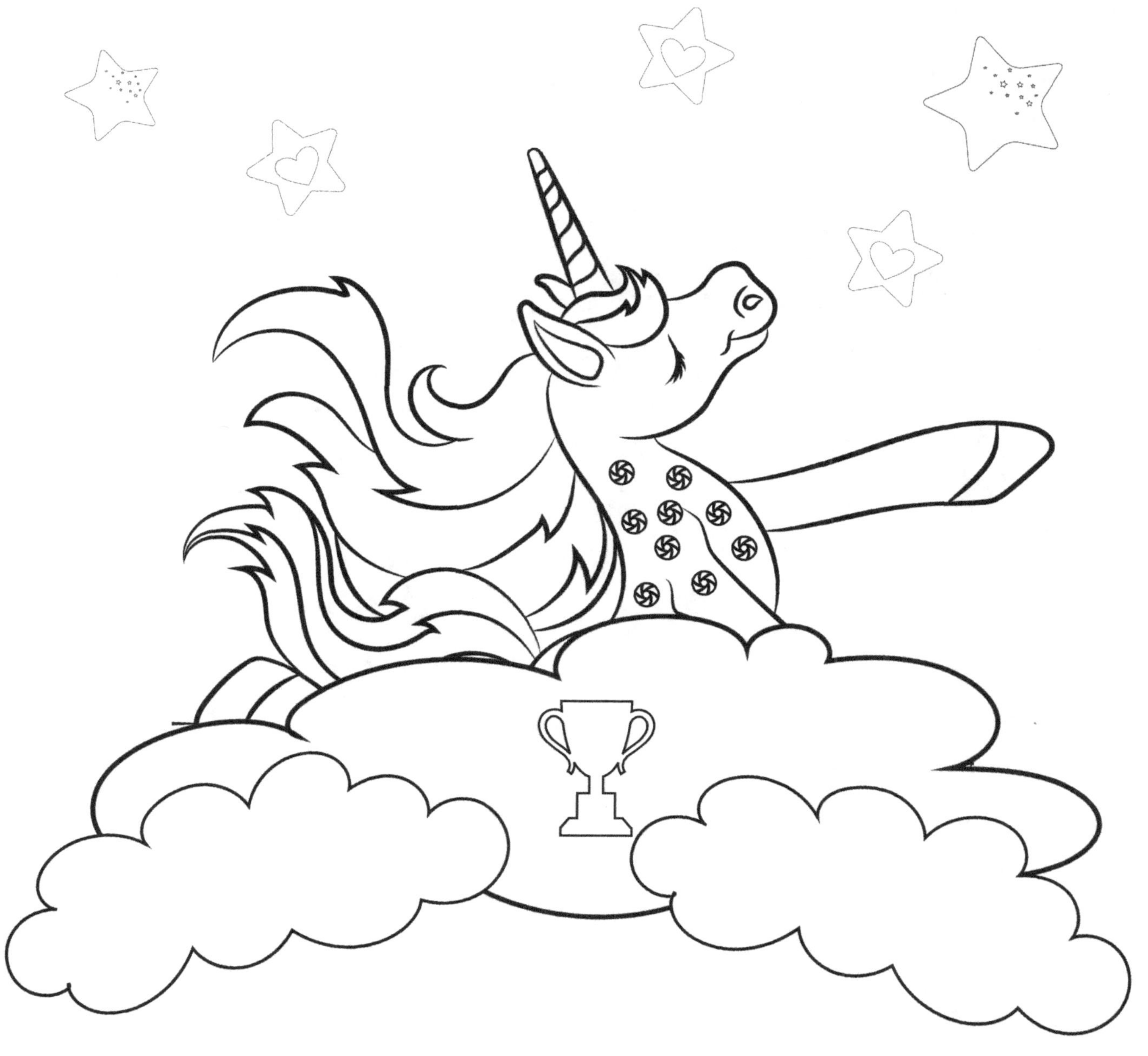

My body helps me to achieve my dreams

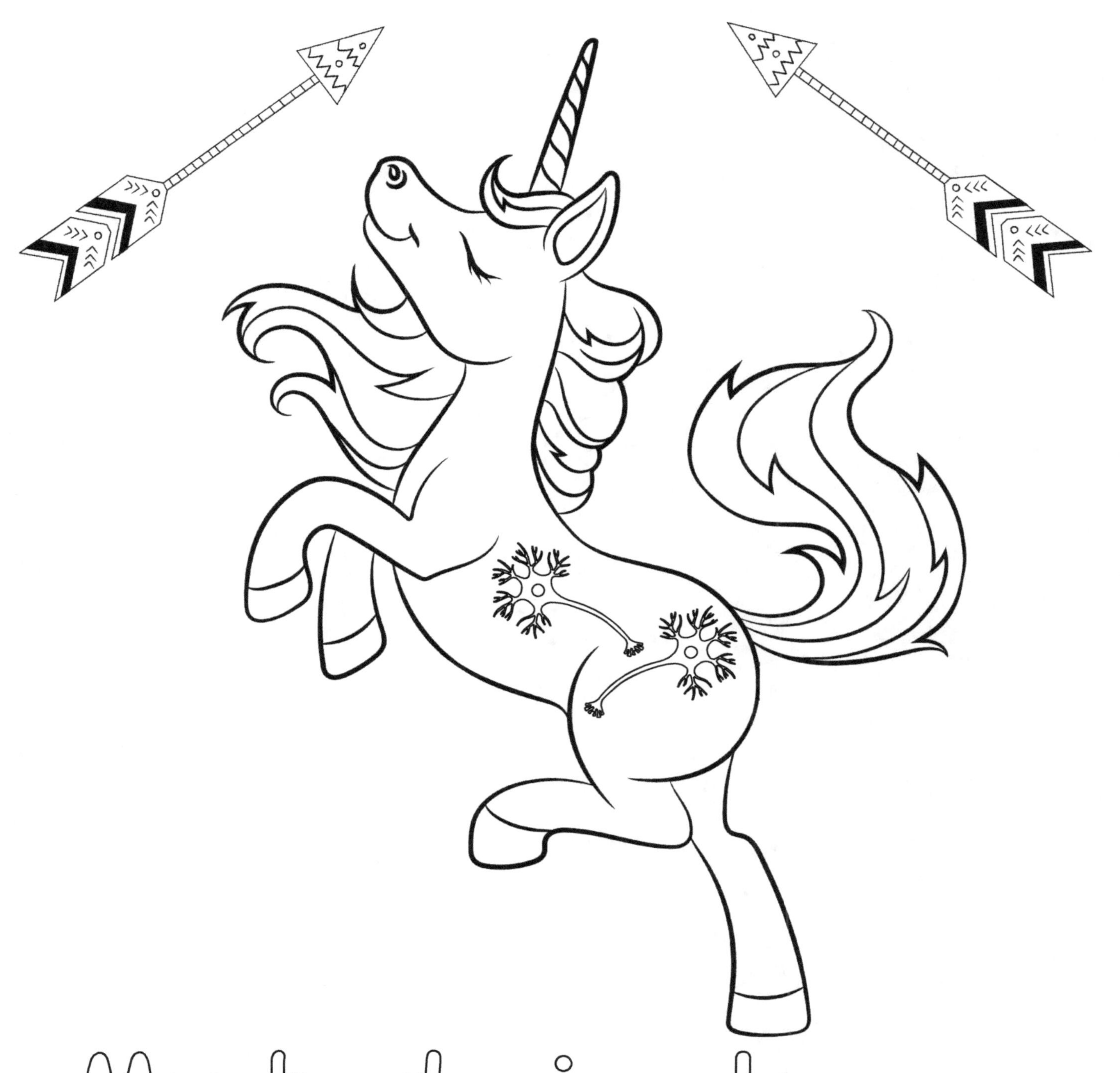

My body is always growing

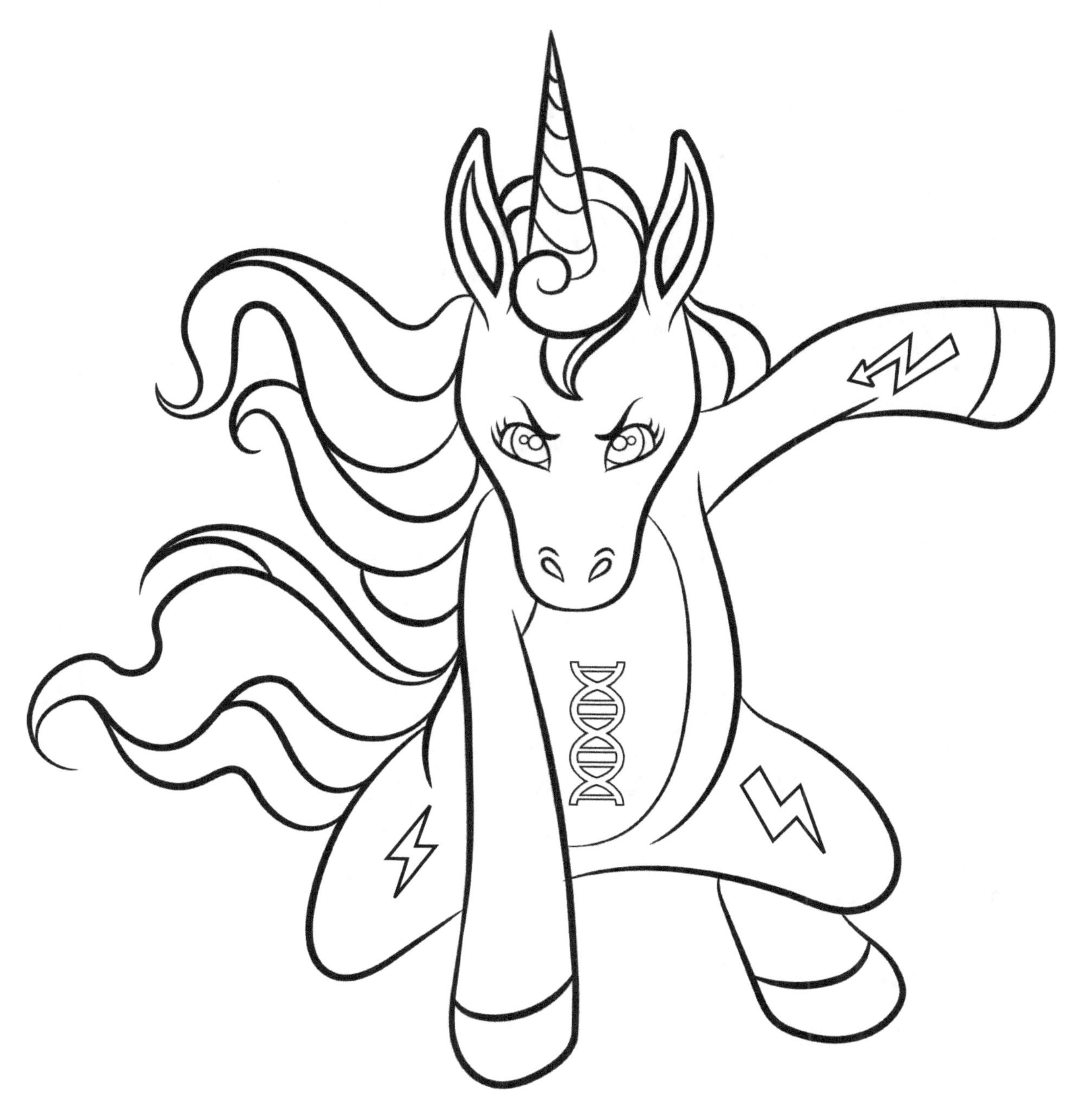

My body is powerful

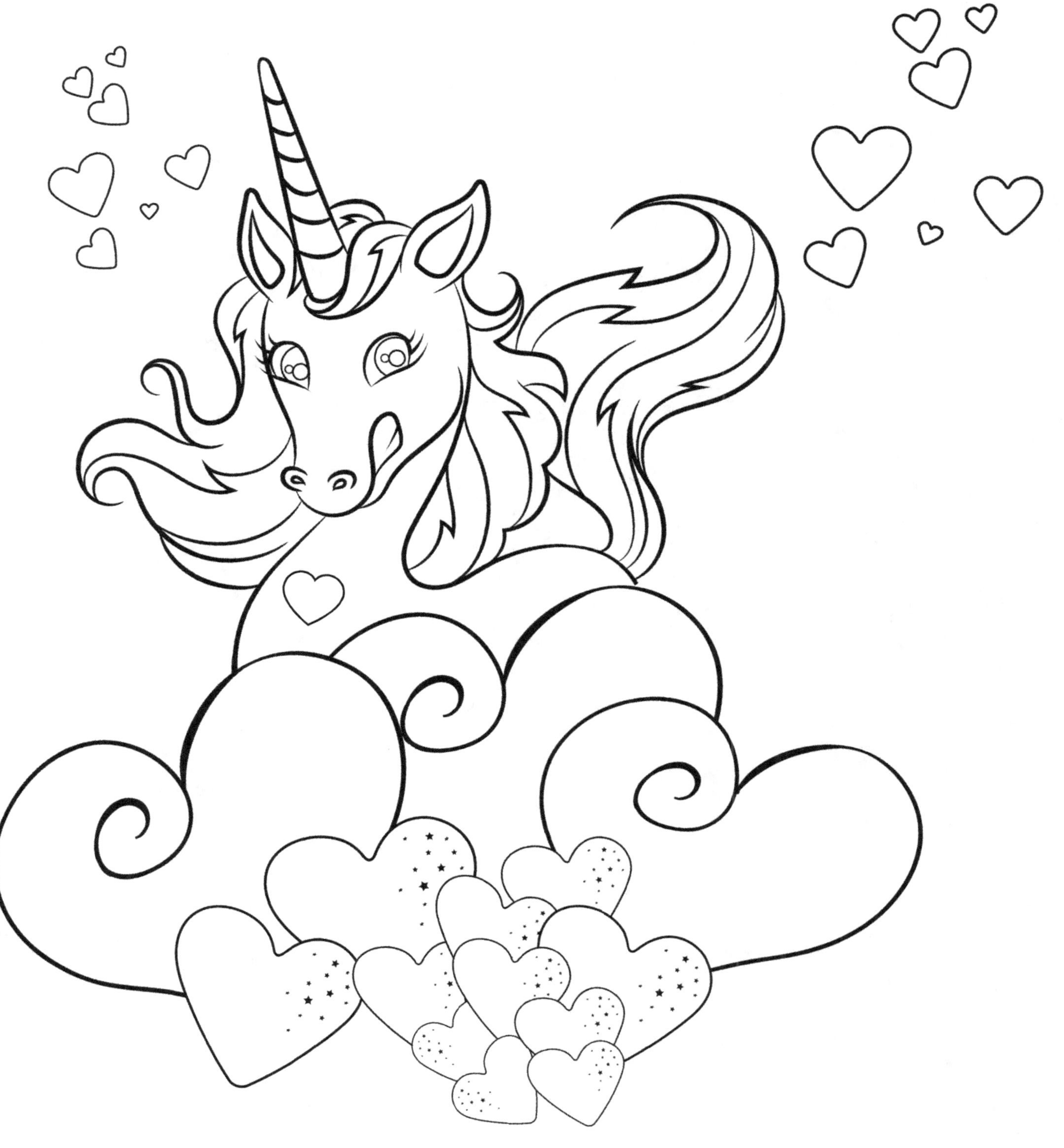

My body is priceless

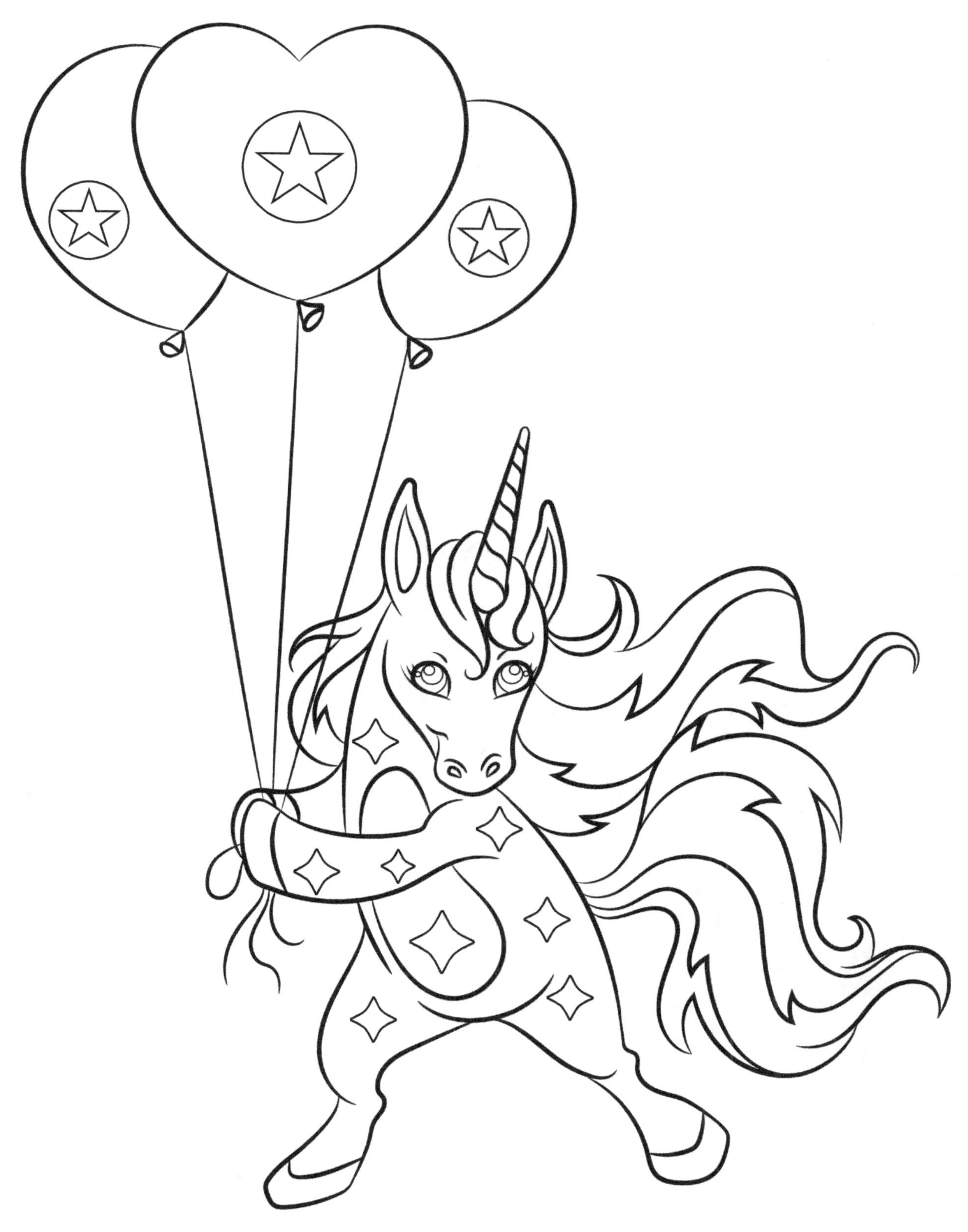

My body is all mine

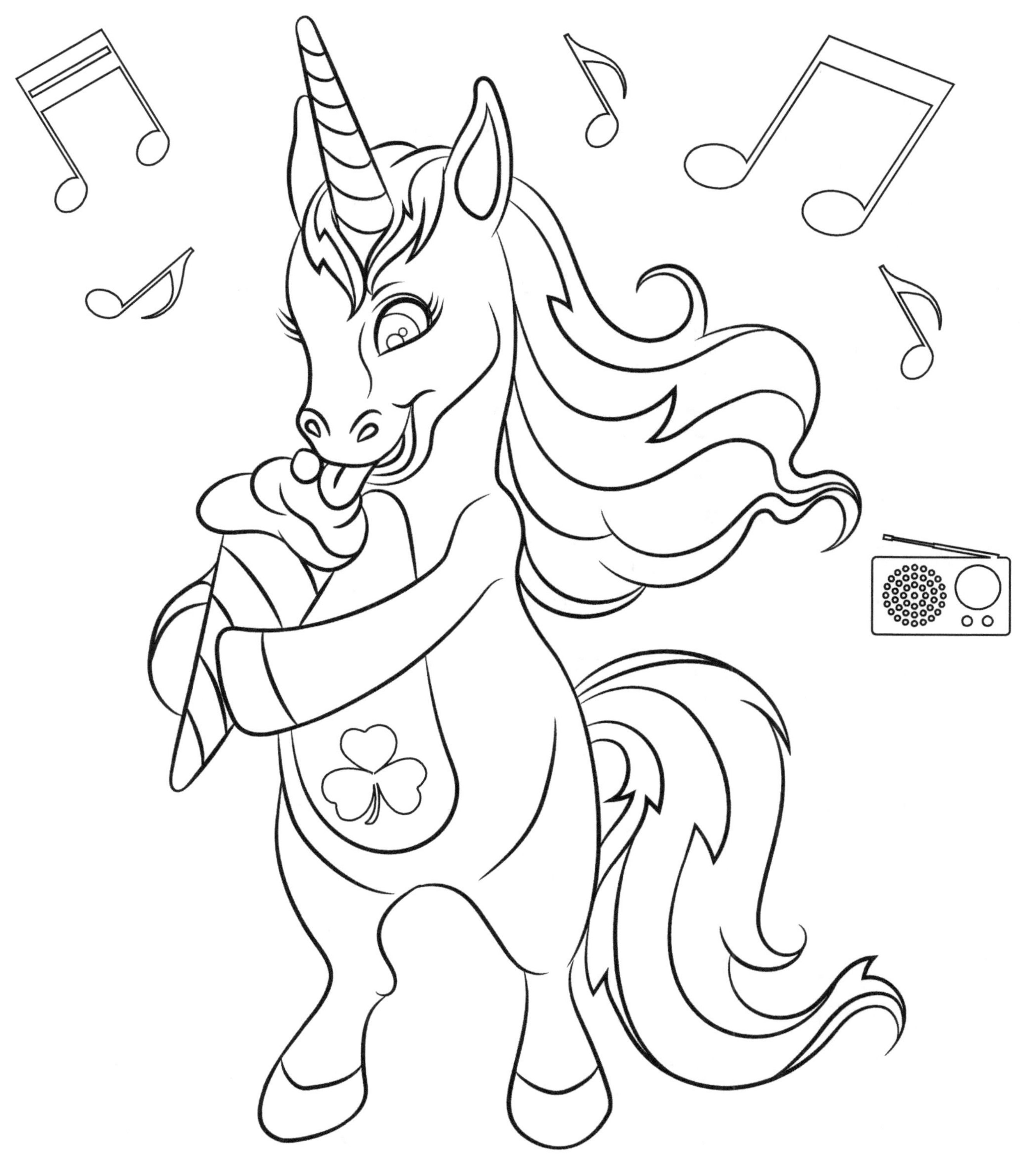

My body allows me to have fun experiences

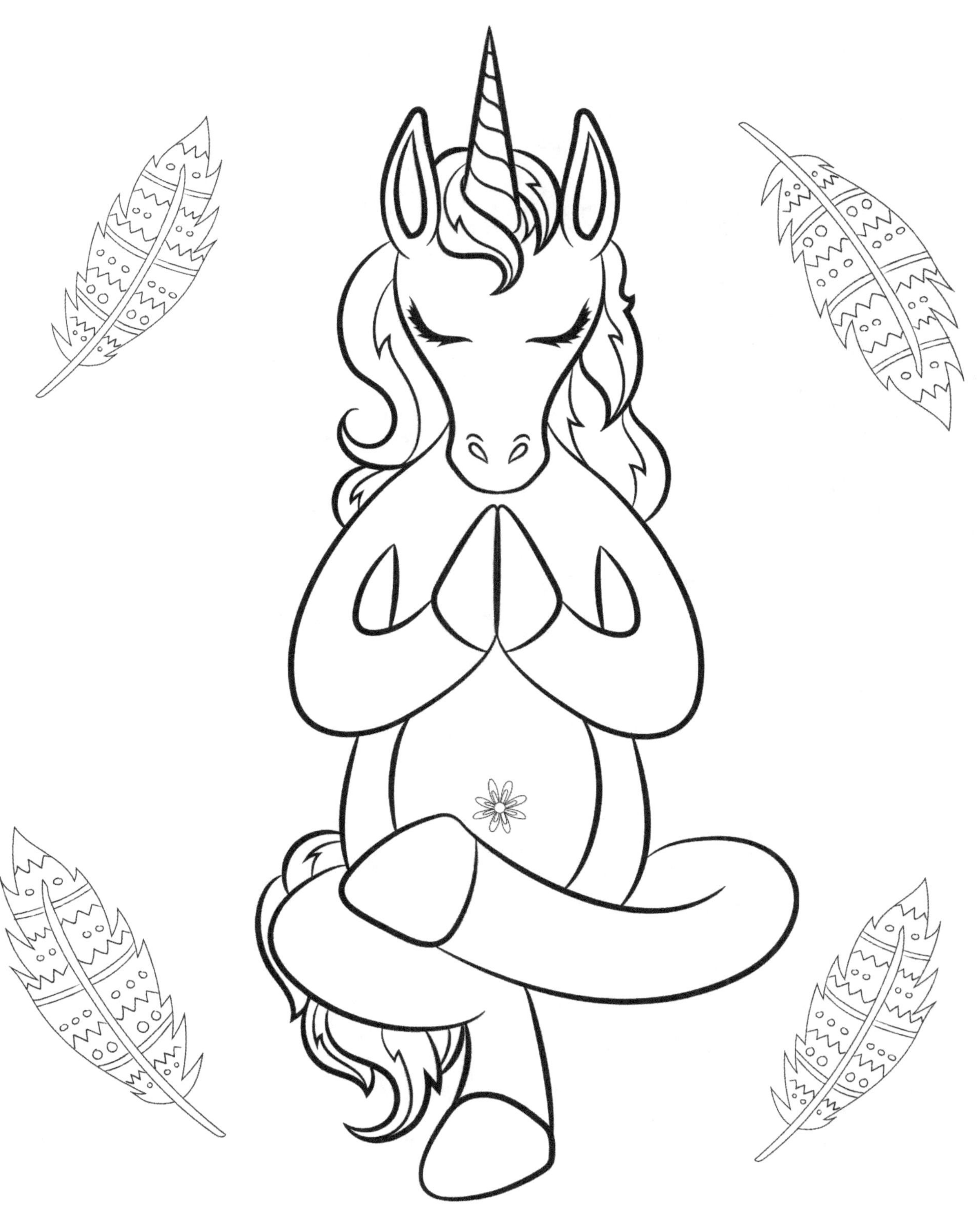

My body can always learn new things

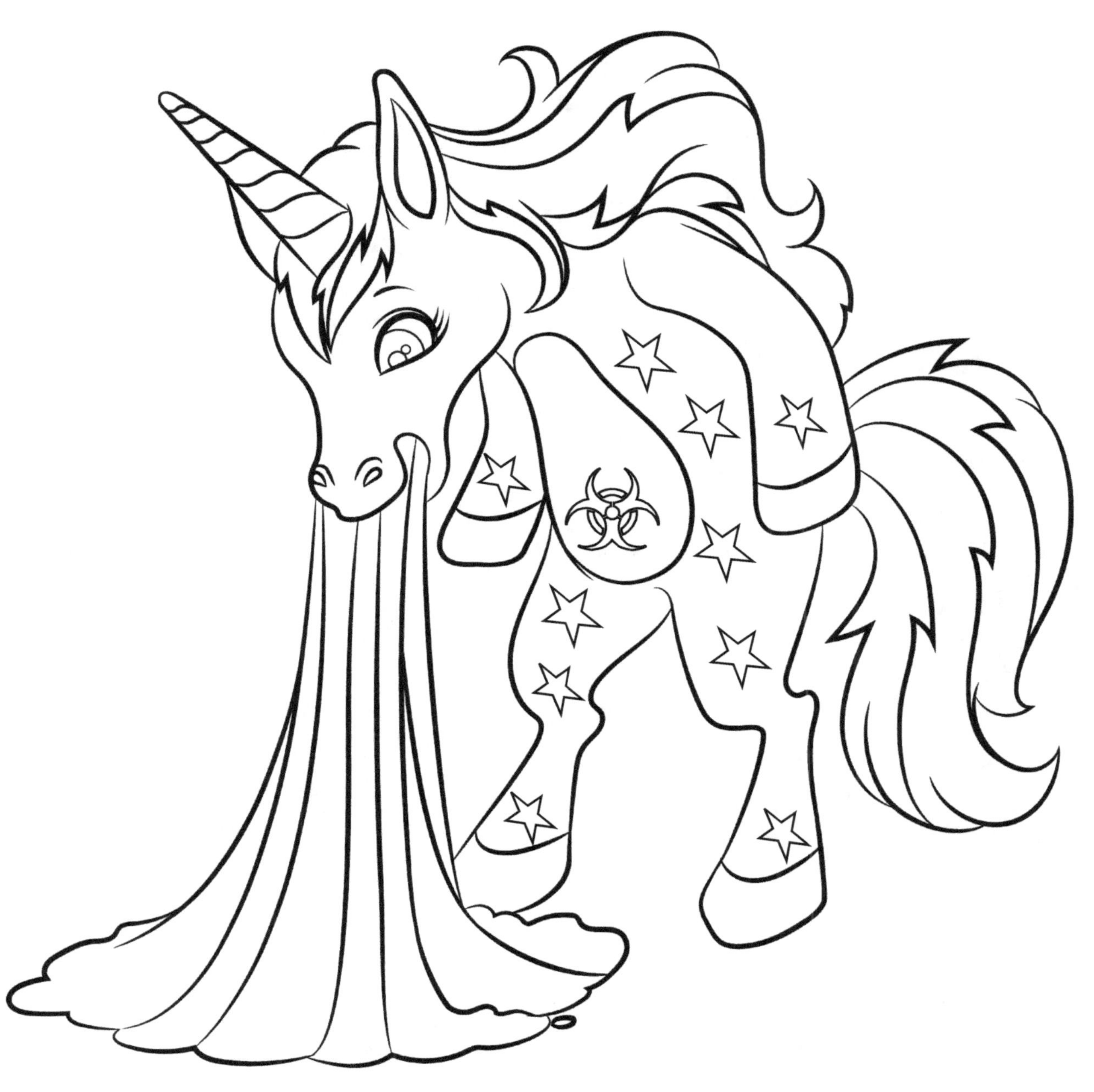

My body is always
working hard to
protect me

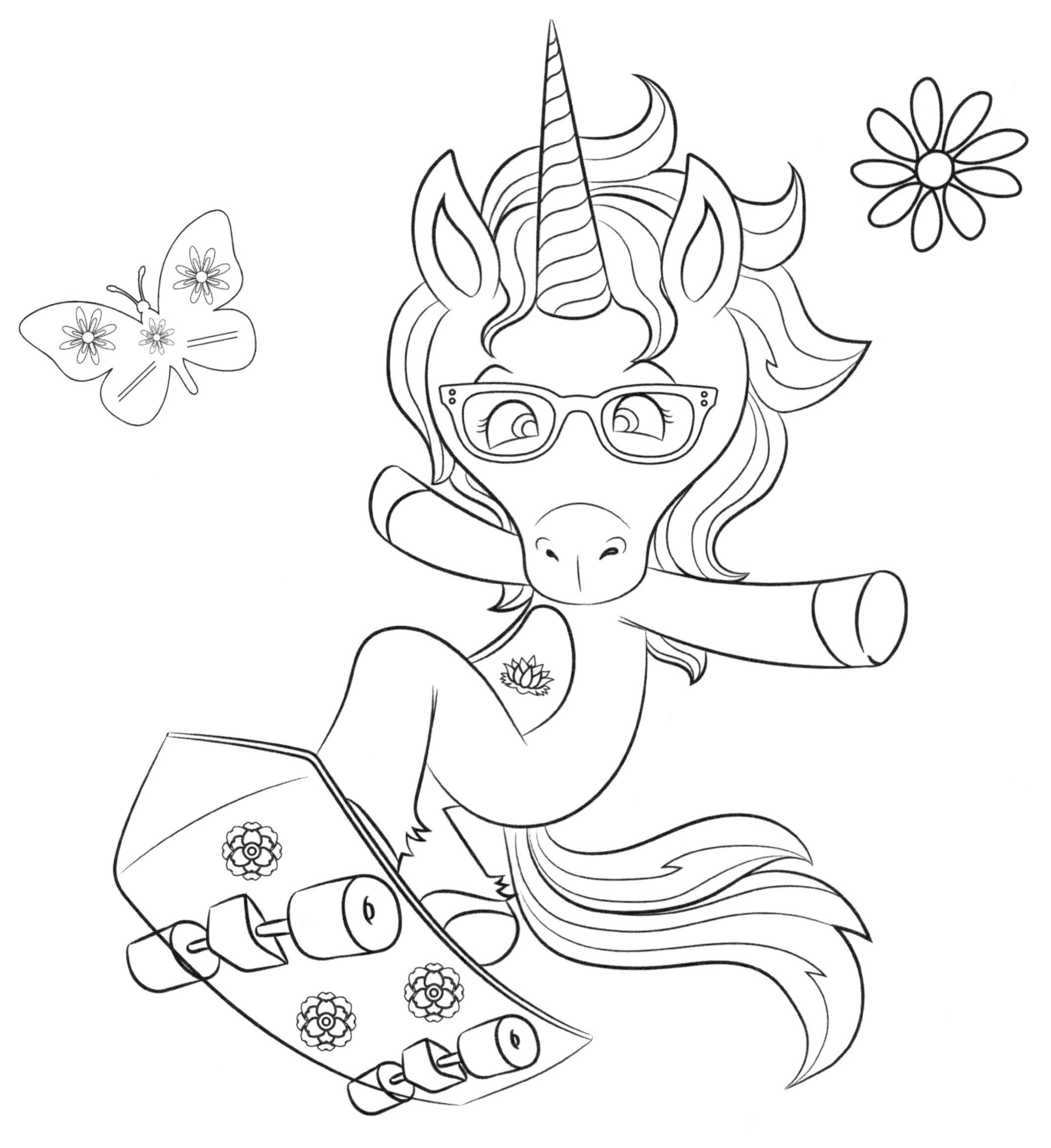

My body is resilient

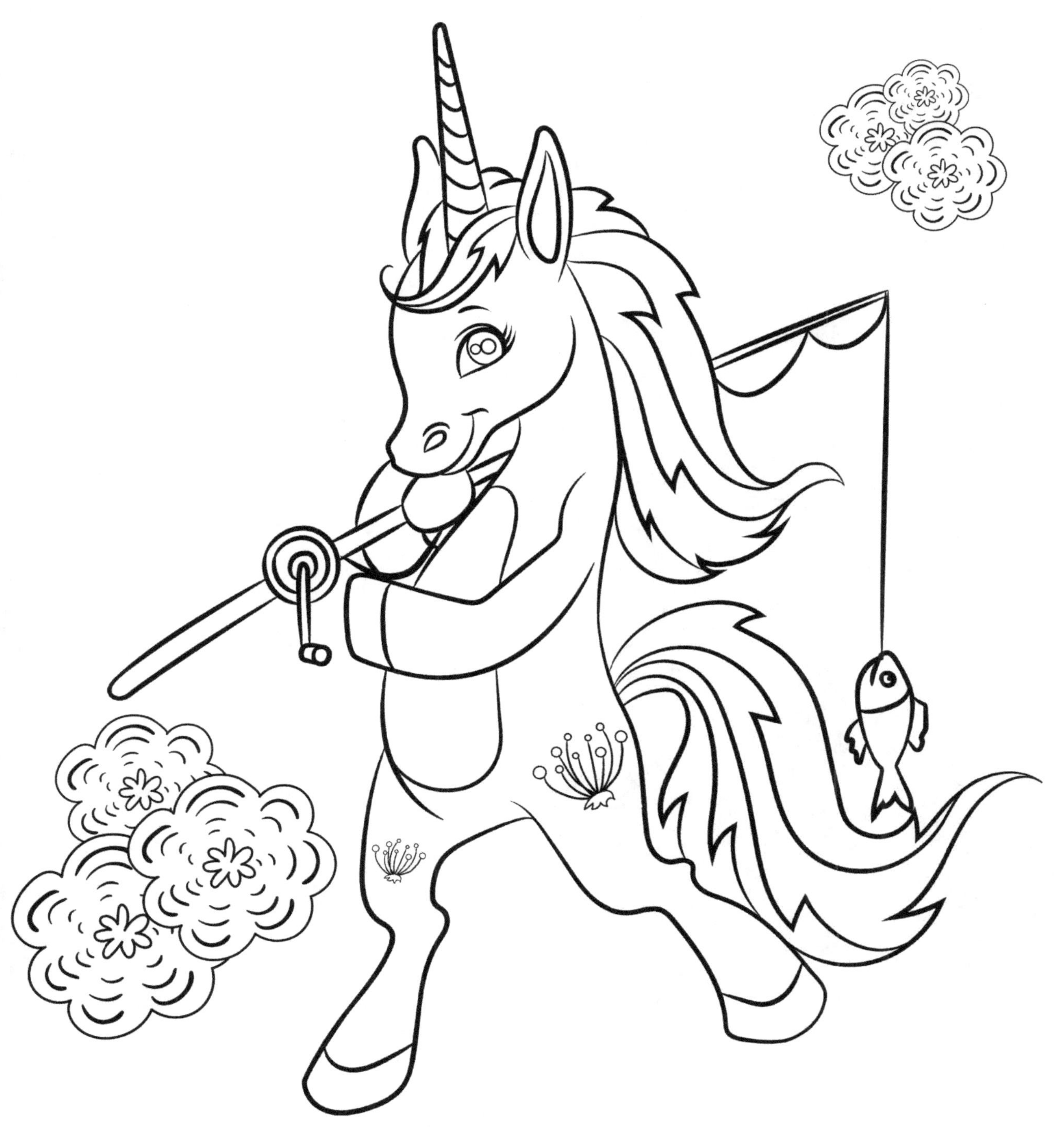

My body likes it when
i try new things

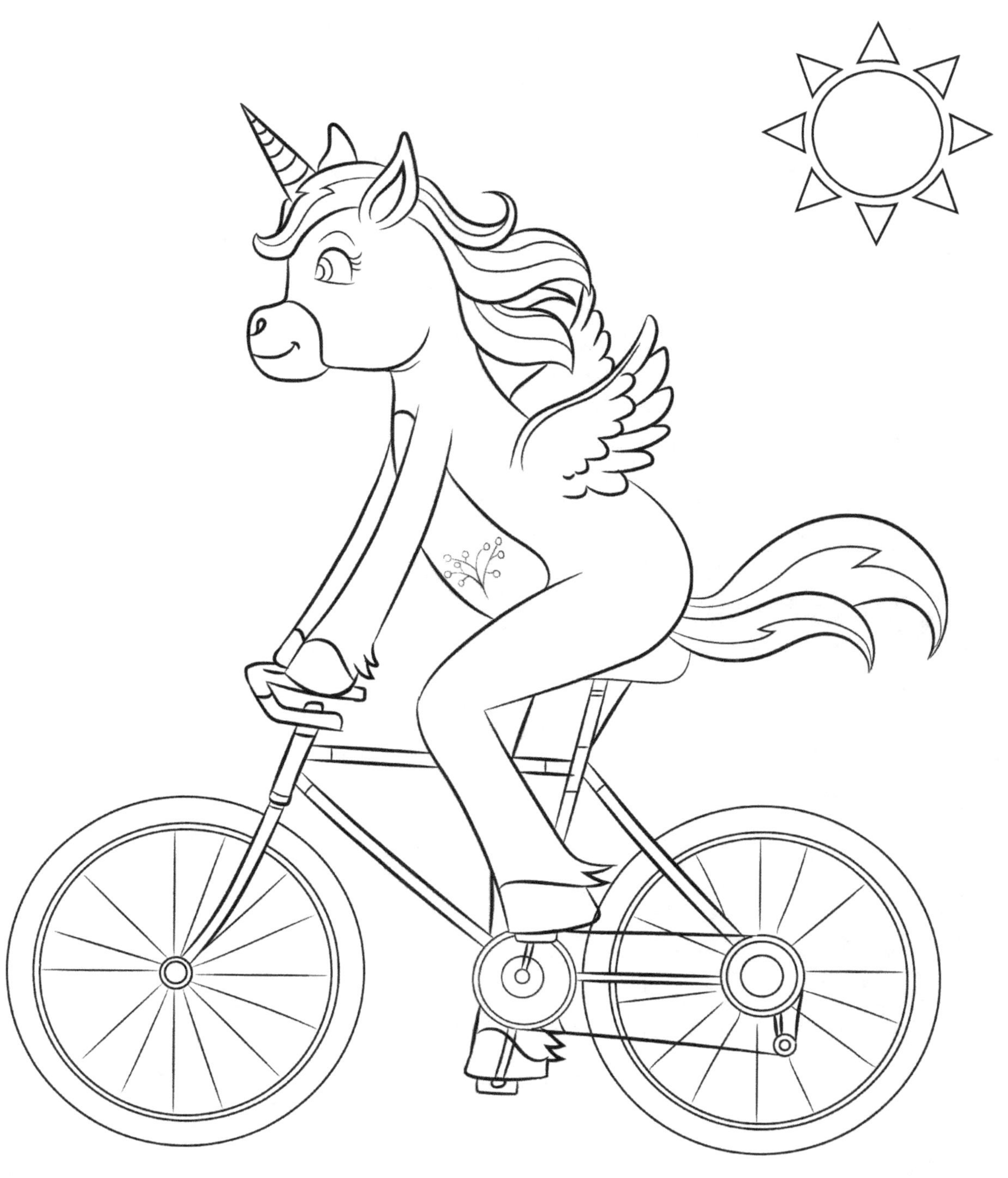

My body likes
to move

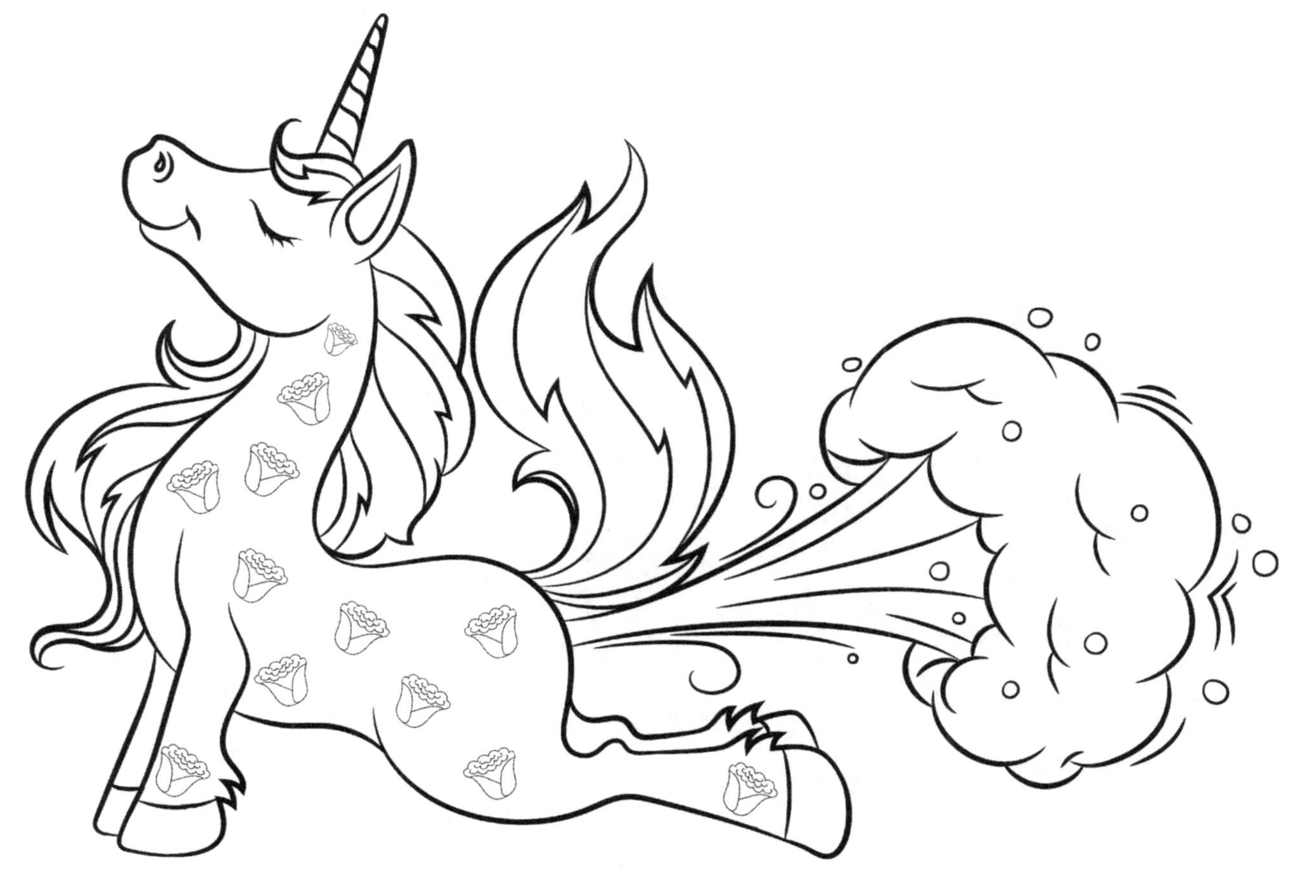

My body is funny
sometimes

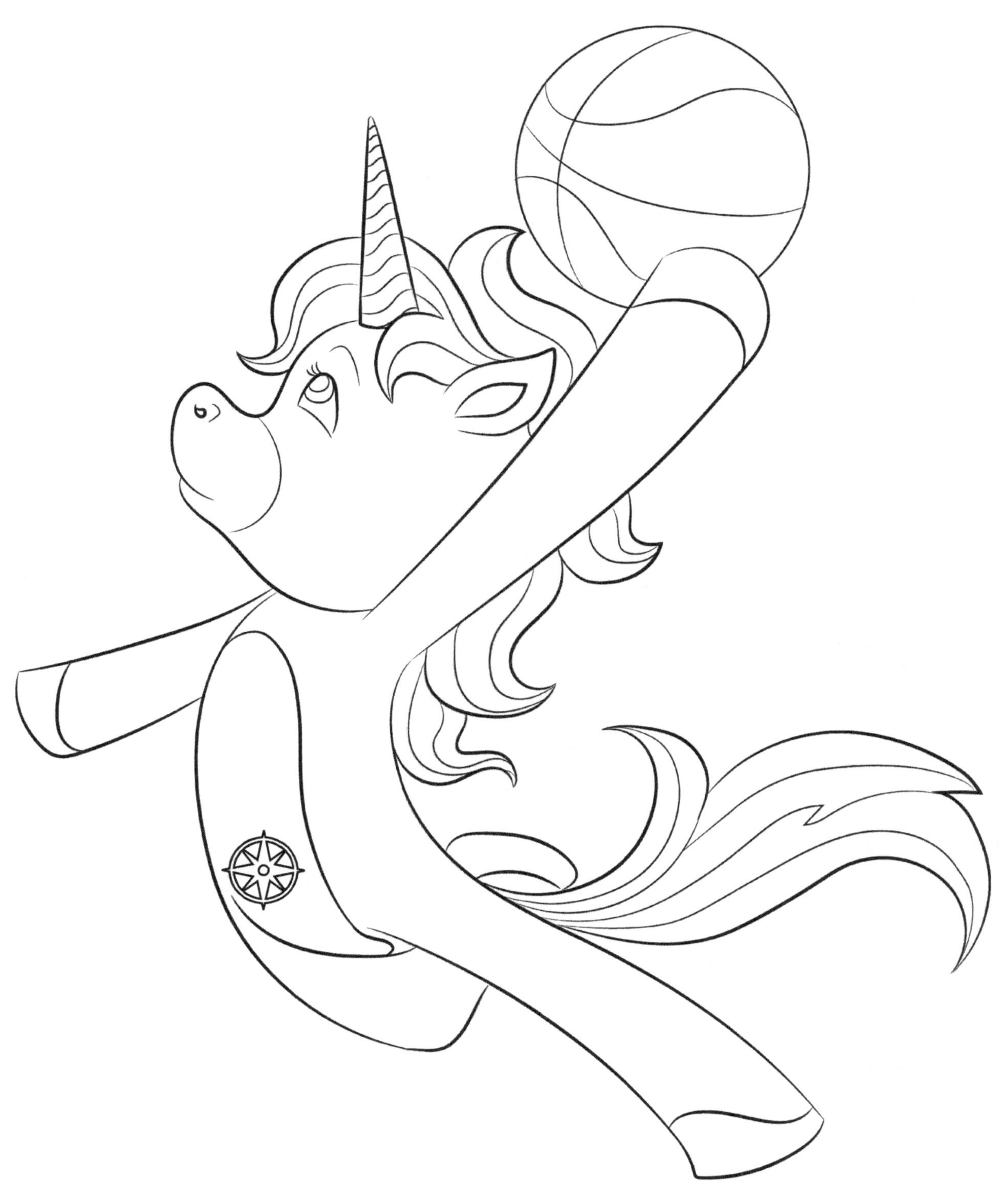

My body is full of
energy

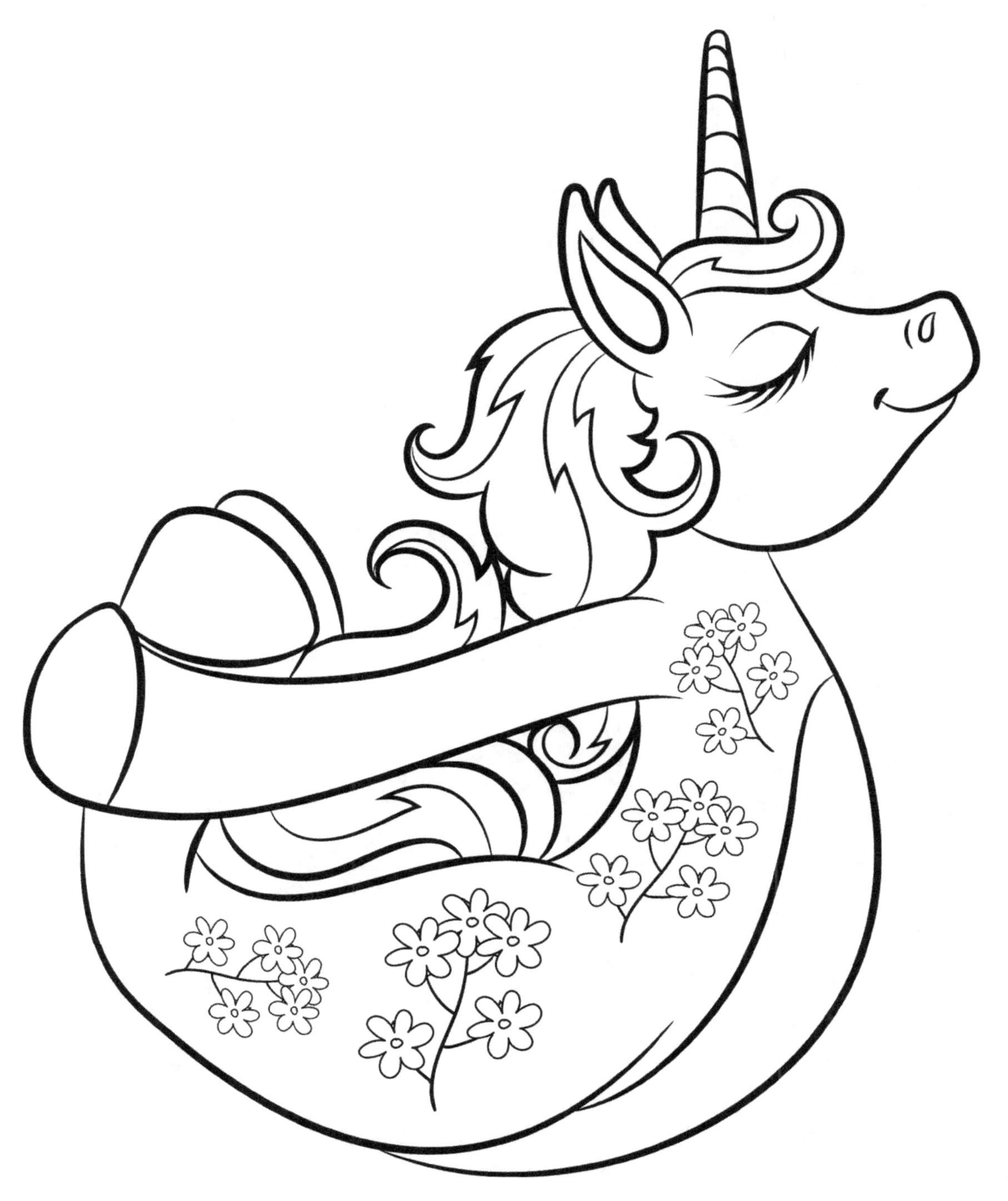

My body is beautiful

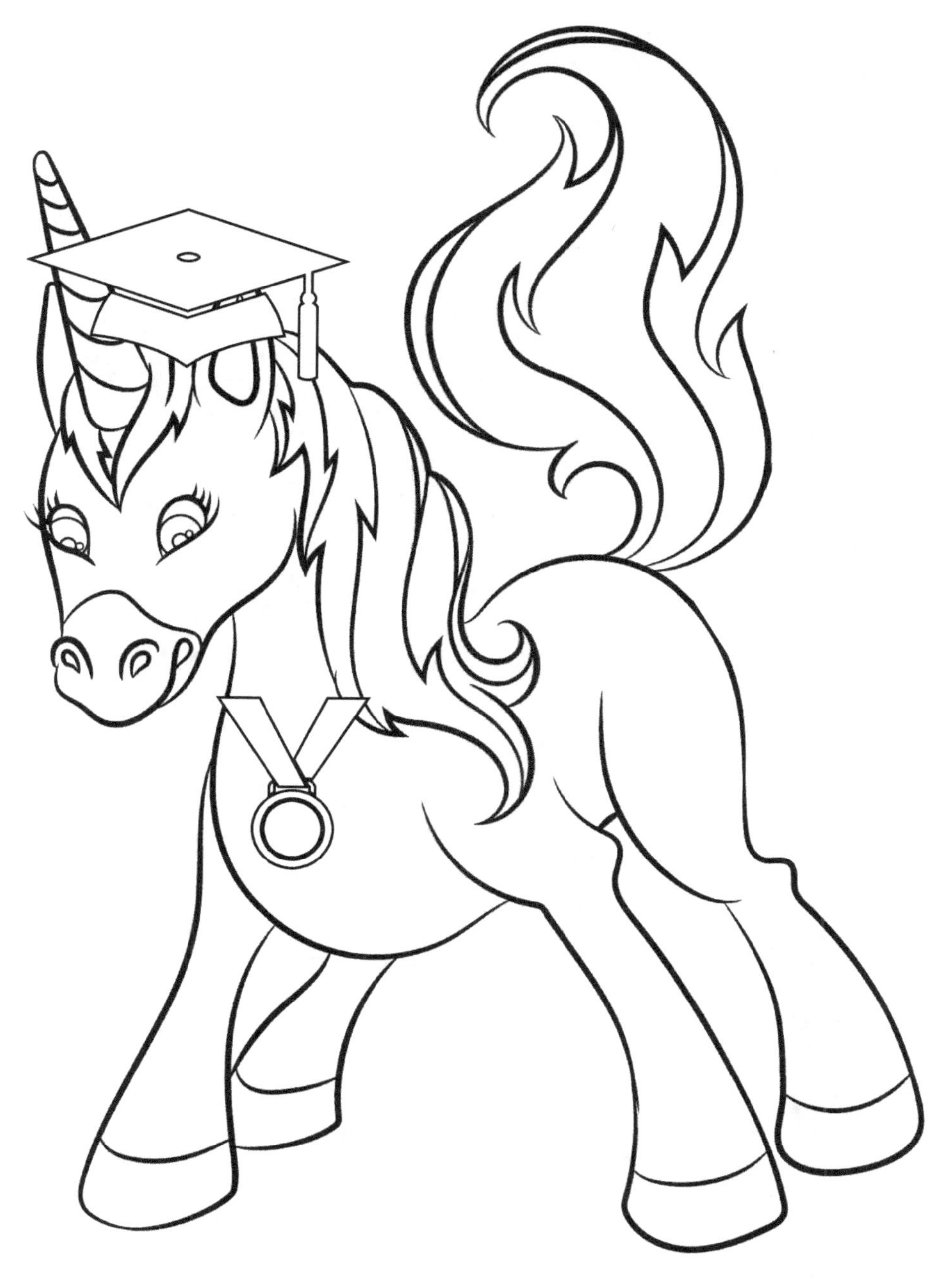

My body is intelligent

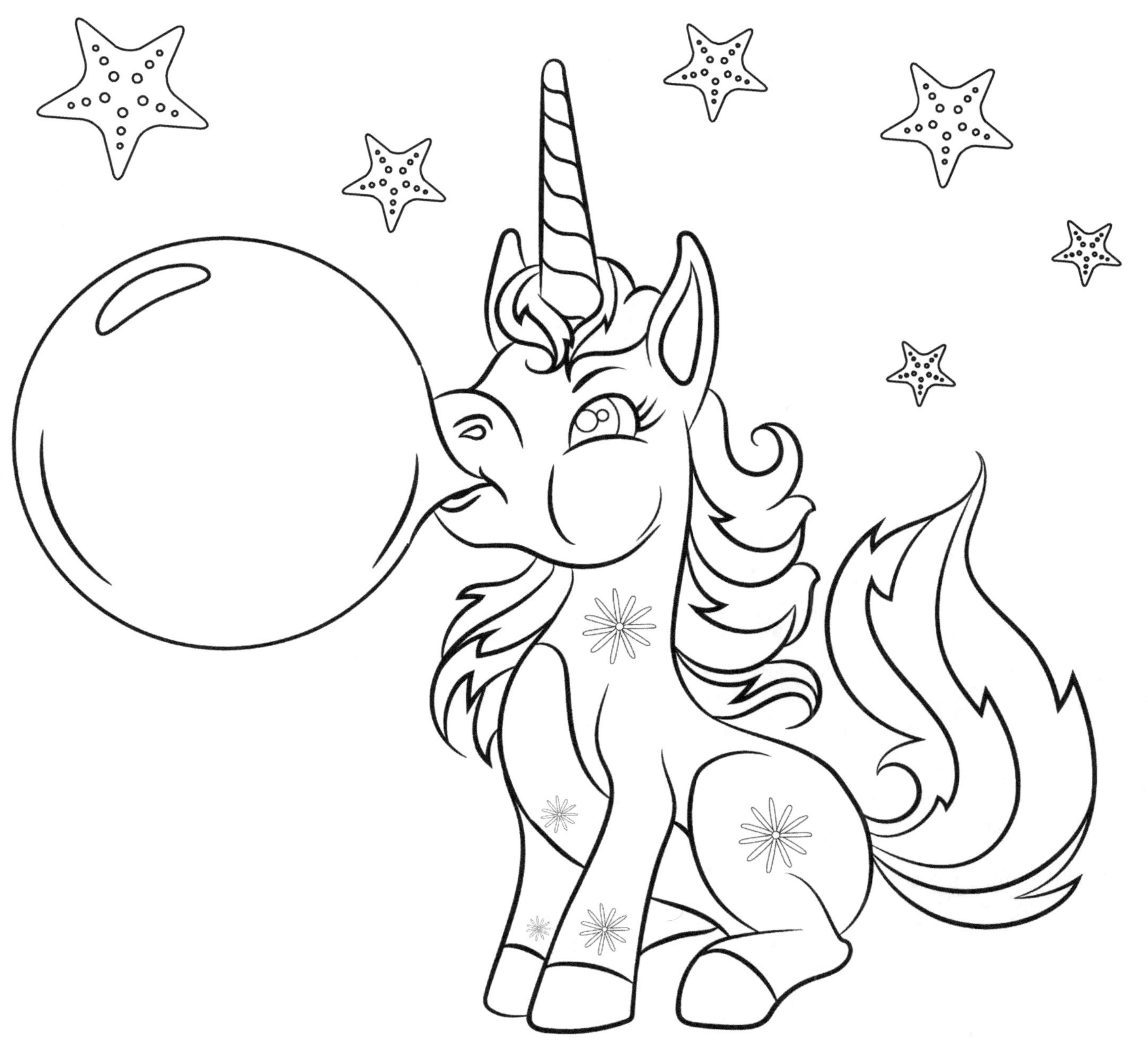
My body can do
wacky things

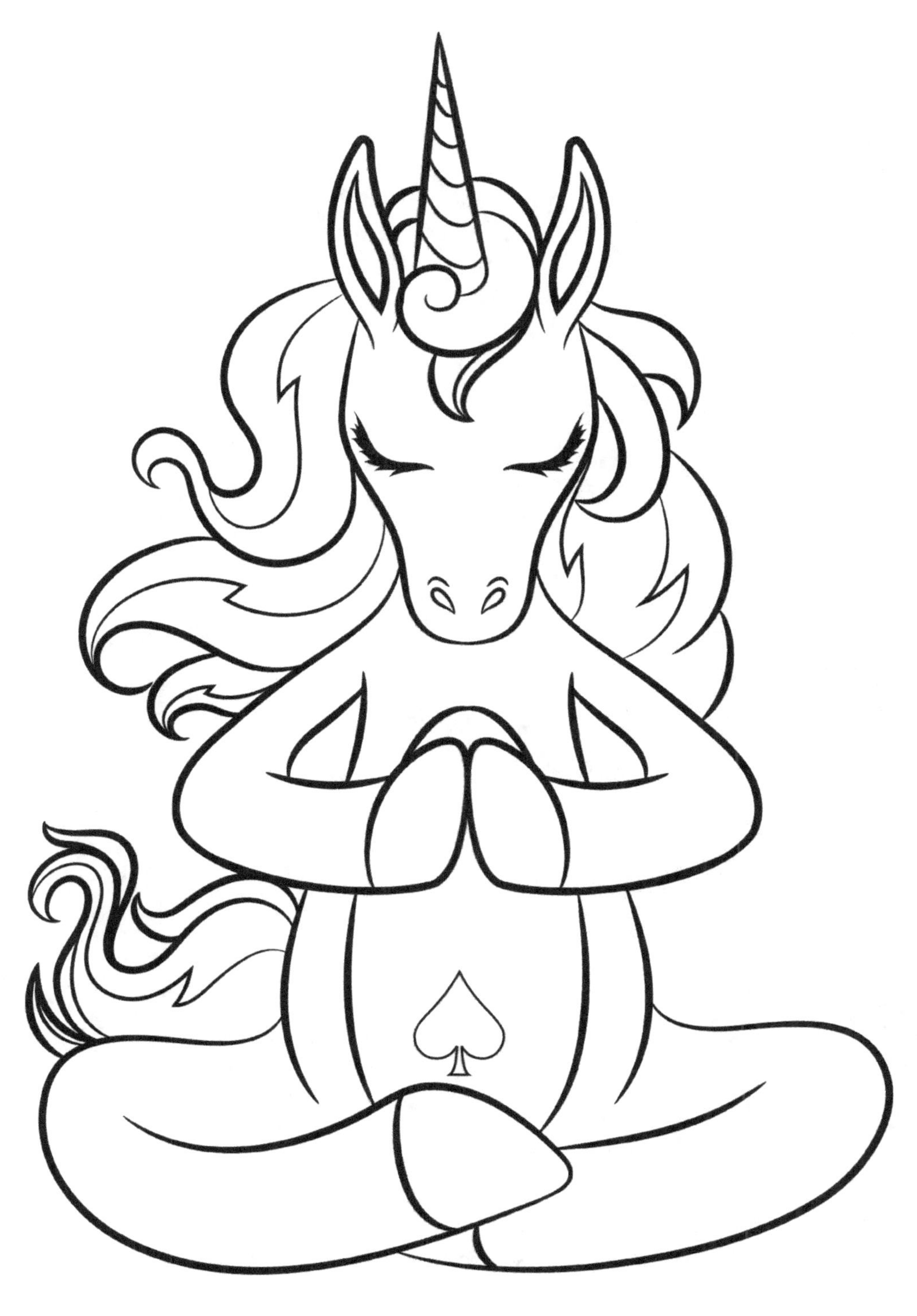

My body deserves
love and respect

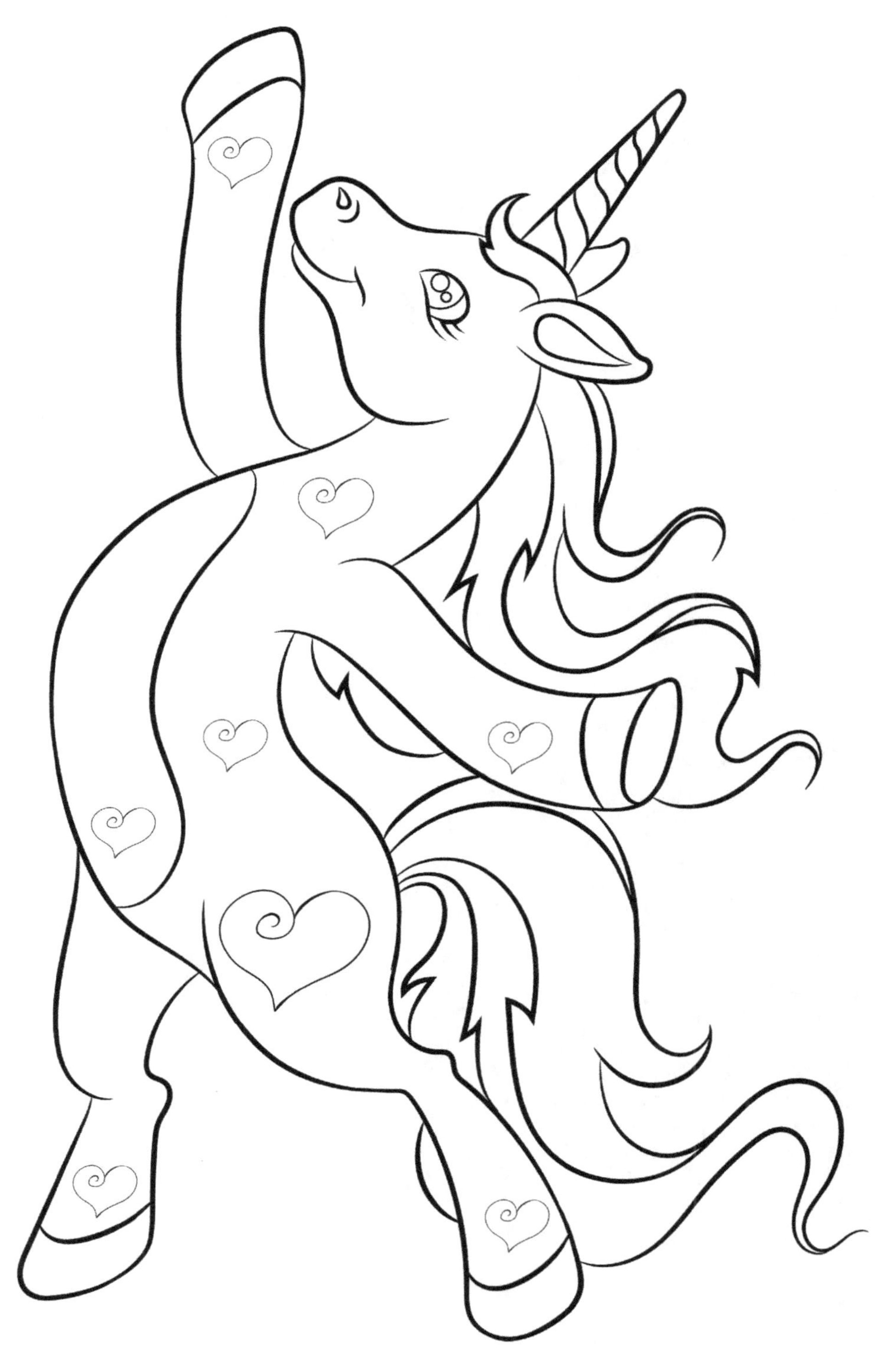

My body is my one
and only